The Psychiatrist's Little Book of Wisdom

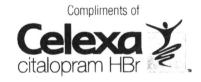
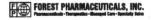

The Psychiatrist's Little Book of Wisdom

350 Tips & Reflections on Clinical Practice and the Art of Communicating

ALLAN PETERKIN, MD

Physicians' Press

Physicians' Press
620 Cherry Street
Royal Oak, MI 48073
Tel: (248) 616-3023
Fax: (248) 616-3003
http://www.physicianspress.com

Printed in the United States of America   ISBN 1-890114-22-7

Preface

Learning to be an empathic and effective psychiatrist and psychotherapist is a lengthy apprenticeship involving many teachers. I owe much to my professors who have guided me in my reading and challenged me in supervision. I am also grateful to my patients who over the years have pushed me to find more of a balance between the art and science of behavioral medicine. **The Psychiatrist's Little Book of Wisdom** grew from these many exchanges. As with all guides containing tips and theoretical directives, caution and proper judgement must be exercised in using these interventions. The brevity of some of these comments is meant to challenge, but does not imply that this work is easy or that it can be abbreviated by clever short-cuts. The clinician must be ethical, well-informed, and able to rigorously justify approaches in a time when actually talking to patients is devalued by some insurers and researchers. I hope this powerful little book of tips and reflections will challenge you to reconsider and affirm what you offer to your patients.

Allan Peterkin, M.D.
Assistant Professor of
Psychiatry and Family Medicine
University of Toronto

THE PATIENT

The Patient

*R*emind your patients that the changes they're making may threaten others in their lives. Some relationships will dissolve, others will deepen.

*C*hallenge tactfully and freely your patients' self-limiting thinking and behaviors. This communicates your belief in their potential and confidence in their strengths.

The Patient

*I*f your patient is stuck in the past, gently remind him: That was then, this is now.

*S*earch for the healthy forms of rebellion your patients used as children or teenagers. These may empower them right now.

*S*elf-esteem is often a vague term or concept. Ask your patients to define what having healthy self-esteem would mean at this stage in their development.

The Patient

*A*re your patients attempting to grow in the wrong soil?
Help them see how natural setting, climate, living
arrangements, work and home environment either nurture
or defeat them.

*R*emind your patients not to berate themselves for old
mistakes, patterns and defenses. They were doing the best
they could with what they had.

*N*ever work with a patient you can't like. Only harm will result.

*R*emind your patients that they can experience more than one feeling at a time. Many people don't realize this.

*F*ind out how your patients tolerate authority figures. This may become a useful focus in therapy.

*F*ocus on your patient's strengths. They are the basis of healing.

The Patient

*F*ind out what your patients were teased about as children. These wounds are usually scarred over but seldom healed.

*W*hen your religious patients insist on being martyrs, remind them that they need a self to be selfless or to attend to the needs of others.

*I*f you've hurt your patient's feelings, find out how and why. Without delay.

❧

*T*he patient involved in litigation or on long-term disability may have too much at stake to get better.

❧

*I*nvite your patients to be as kind to themselves as they are to their best friends.

The Patient

*H*elp your patients see that as people they are so much more than their pasts and their current level of distress.

*P*atients who had a mentally ill parent will require much reassurance that they are neither weak nor crazy.

*F*ind out which dreams your patients have given up on.

The Patient

"*N*o man is an island." Encourage your patients to develop a sense of belonging through community involvement.

❧

*H*ave your patients ask themselves three questions when overwhelmed: 1) What am I feeling? 2) What do I want? and 3) What can I do about it?

The Patient

*I*t feels better for the therapist to be idealized than devalued, but they both speak of the same thing: narcissistic injury.

*I*f your patient is rambling or vague, tactfully point it out. You may be the first to dare to do so.

*I*f your patients' symptoms represent a compromise, what are their options?

The Patient

*F*ind out about your patient's best friend now and in childhood. Seek out healthy signs of generosity, love, altruism, and caring. Help your patient to build on these feelings.

*M*uch of your patient's life is spent in school or work. Remember to ask about social functioning as well as performance in these settings.

*R*emember that your patients
may cling to your diagnosis
as an excuse <u>not</u> to get
better.

The Patient

*E*xplore with your patients the ways their workplace mirrors their family dynamics. What familiar role are they playing?

*D*on't be surprised when a patient flees from you or despises you for being kind. Kindness may be foreign and terrifying.

The Patient

*W*hat gifts or talents are your patients concealing, what light are they hiding under a bushel?

*D*on't allow your patients to oversubscribe to any one identity: victim, AIDS survivor, cancer patient, mother, professional. They are selling themselves short.

*A*sk your obsessive client: What's so great about control?

The Patient

*R*emind your patients that memory is poetic—prone to imagination, hearsay, suggestion, distortion. What feels true is only partly so.

*I*nvite your patients to define compassion. Ask them to look for evidence of it in their relationships with themselves and with others.

*F*ind out how much your patients like and care for their bodies.

The Patient

*A*sk your patients to teach you about their culture and community, even if you think you know all about it. You may both learn something as a result of this new scrutiny.

*I*f your patient wants a motto, consider the Prayer of St. Francis: Grant me the strength to change the things I can, the courage to face those I can't, and the wisdom to know the difference.

The Patient

Always ask about past experiences with psychotherapy—how your patient experienced the previous therapist, the approach and termination process. Comparisons and contamination from old work are inevitable. Be prepared to address them.

Your first goal is to teach your patients how to observe themselves in new ways: thoughts, feelings, interactions with others, and behaviors must be noted, remembered, recorded. Invite them to merely observe and not to judge.

The Patient

*F*ind out how your patients have coped with previous crises. This will help them build on old strengths and coping skills.

*A*sk your patients about secret habits, rituals, compulsions. They may reveal much.

*T*each your patients to titrate anger: neither too little nor too much, as required by each situation.

The Patient

*E*ncourage your patients to follow intuitions, to "go with their gut." They may experience a breakthrough.

*C*ould your patient be gay or bisexual? Why don't you know?

*H*ave your patients keep records of all negative, critical thoughts or self-depreciations for one whole day. It will help you and your patients see what you're up against.

THE THERAPIST

Warning: Your own narrow world vision may limit your patient's gains.

Never accept a patient you don't like or can't help just for the money. If you do so, acknowledge what that makes you.

Why would you dismiss discussing dreams if they mean something to your client?

The Therapist

Strive to remain open to new understanding and experience.

It's good for you to cross disciplines, techniques, and theories. If you practice only adult individual therapy, formulate your case from a couple-, child-, family-, or group-therapy point of view. Take a workshop in a treatment modality you know little about.

The Therapist

When is your lunch break? When is your next holiday? When is your next sabbatical? When will you know it's time to quit doing therapy?

❧

Are you setting up a patient you don't like to fire you?

❧

When working with a traumatized patient, avoid re-enacting the role of rescuer, perpetrator or victim.

*F*our options for the "stuck" therapist:
1) Get supervision
2) Seek personal therapy
3) Take a holiday
4) Retire

The Therapist

*L*earn to listen with openness and a free-floating attention, so that you can discern larger trends and themes amidst all the details.

*Y*ou have no right to give into boredom in a session. Use the boredom to help your patient.

*A*re you avoiding the topics of sex, and death and dying in your work?

Set limits but model flexibility.

*W*hat are your own ambitions for your patients? What limitations have you placed on them? How do these differ from their own? From their parents?

*O*n occasion, you may fall asleep or tune right out during a patient's session. Don't pretend you didn't. Just apologize.

*F*ind ways to nurture your soul or this work will deplete you.

The Therapist

What is your own Achilles' heel as a person and as a therapist? Money? Social status? Childlessness? Loneliness? Class? Race? Physical or mental illness?

Sadism. Sarcasm. Envy. Lust. Jealousy. Romantic love. Competition. Guilt. Arrogance. Superiority. Rage. Idealization. Neediness. Fear. Intimidation. Passivity. Longing. Grief. Impatience. Degradation. Be prepared to recognize and understand these traits in yourself as you work with patients.

*T*he depth achieved in
therapy is inversely
proportional to
the therapist's fears.

Watch for counter-transference red flags: forgetting names, dates, appointments.

❦

When you tune out in a session, where do you go? Learn to use that place and those thoughts to deepen your understanding of your patient and of your process with him.

❦

Are you afraid of letting your patient go?

Are you a "one note" therapist? Do you respond only to some material or feelings your patients bring but ignore the rest?

The Therapist

*E*mpathy is not a quality you can turn on and off in between sessions. How kind are you to your colleagues, students and staff? To those in your life outside the office?

*Y*ou don't have to be a perfect therapist. You have to be "good enough."

*W*rite a profile of patients who drop out from your practice. What do they reveal about you and your method?

*W*hich patients do you refuse to treat? What do they reveal about you?

*B*efore giving an Axis II personality disorder diagnosis, ensure that you don't merely dislike the patient.

*T*here is nothing wrong with using your title unless your patient would be more comfortable calling you something else.

Watch for the times you
feel heroic or paralyzed.

Consider doing pro bono or volunteer work for an under-serviced community, group or population. Your skills will be challenged and your sense of purpose enhanced.

Each time you are about to make an exception for a client ask yourself why. Sometimes bending the rules is about softening boundaries, altering the frame, liking a patient too much, or trying too hard to please.

The Therapist

*B*ecome a teacher or psychotherapy supervisor. It keeps you sharper longer.

❦

*O*ff-call means off-call. You gave at the office. Don't take the job home.

❦

*D*on't let yourself be cast as an authority figure, especially if you like to be one.

*D*on't be married to your theory. Offer what the client needs or refer them on.

The Therapist

*Y*ou only think you've worked through your blind spots.
New ones develop all the time.

*B*oundary violations—sexual, financial, social—develop
insidiously over time. Don't fool yourself into thinking it
could never happen to you. If something doesn't feel right
early on, it probably isn't.

*I*f you think your job is only to prescribe medications, read this book twice.

The Therapist

*B*eware of pseudo-insight, pseudo-gains, pseudo-work. These make you a pseudo-therapist.

❧

*D*espite what you think, your patients know as much about your quirks as you do about their quirks.

❧

*W*ould you care as much if you were paid less?

*I*f you've heard it all before,
you're not listening.

The Therapist

$\mathcal{N}$ever undermine an approach that may help your patient. In this day and age, you have no right to be either "anti- drug" or "anti-therapy."

$\mathcal{K}$nowing what you know now, write an update or thank-you note to your own previous therapist. Have you and your method evolved?

The Therapist

*F*irst do no harm. We all have hang-ups regarding sexuality, political or religious ideation. It is your duty not to judge your patients or impose these views. If you run into conflict, seek out supervision or refer the patient to another therapist.

*Y*ou have a moral and often legal duty to report unethical, incompetent or harmful colleagues. Consult your licensing body for guidelines and advice.

$\mathcal{D}$o not do this work if you
are friendless.

*S*elf-reveal selectively if it will help the therapy. Ask yourself whether the information is really of use to the patient in that moment, or an unburdening for you.

*O*nly discuss a patient with a colleague if the goal is learning or confidential ventilation on your part. Don't vent your spleen or act out your own countertransference in a careless, harmful fashion.

*P*oor compliance is usually the doctor's fault. You have not educated, persuaded or dispelled fears enough.

The Therapist

*D*on't sign on too quickly to new treatments, trends or fad therapies. Be rigorous in your evaluation of these.

*Y*ou will someday cry with a patient. Allow this to happen.

*K*now when to say, "I don't think I'm the one to help you. I'll help you to find someone else."

*E*xperience your own conversions, revelations and epiphanies on your own time, not in your patient's hour.

*F*lip your theories and concepts on their head. For example, what if "repetition compulsion" were an attempt at learning or mastery? How would that change your work with the client?

*D*on't take being fired personally, and don't resign too easily. Gently interpret your patient's fear and resistance and keep at it.

The Therapist

*A*lways tell the truth. Patients seem to know when you're fudging, rationalizing, or protecting them.

*R*ecognize when you are in danger. Know the signs of potential violence and how to protect yourself, your staff and your family.

*O*ne day, despite your best efforts, a patient may commit suicide. Reflect carefully, and speak to someone kind.

$\mathcal{K}$eep in touch with new ideas and trends in therapy. Go to rounds, seminars and retreats.

❦

$\mathcal{Y}$ou can attend your patient's funeral if you want to.

❦

$\mathcal{W}$hen you get annoyed with patients, remember: The grandiose feel so small, the paranoid so afraid and the histrionic so ignored.

The Therapist

Your partner, friends and kids didn't ask you to be a shrink. Don't take it out on them!

Injury brought you to this work. This work can bring you injury. Take care of yourself.

*B*e a team player. Acknowledge and

assist the work of others.

The Therapist

$\mathcal{R}$ate yourself 1 - 10 on the following traits:

Empathy	___	Warmth	___
Respect	___	Capacity to confront	___
Genuineness	___	Personal integrity	___
Common sense	___	Capacity to	
Immediacy	___	self-disclose	___
("here and now" emphasis)		Openness to learn	___

Your score = ___ / 100

*W*rite your definition of empathy here:

_____.

❦

*Y*ou wouldn't drive a car if you were too exhausted, upset or distracted. So don't do therapy at those times.

You are a sponge for grief and rage. Wring yourself out regularly.

THE PROCESS

The Process

*D*o you have an unseen co-therapist? Sometimes patients "tell all" about therapy to a third party in order to diminish the intensity of their sessions. Invite your patient to process the work primarily with you.

*C*larify your patient's principle goal. Is it intrapsychic (enhancing self-esteem, grieving, repairing injury) or interpersonal (enhancing relationships)? Both may coexist but one will usually predominate.

$\mathcal{M}$ake a point of considering compassionately your patients' impact on the people in their lives.

The Process

*A*sk your patients to describe what exactly it is that you do.   You may be surprised.

❧

*Y*ou may have to push the intellectualizer into feeling.

❧

*I*nquire regularly about risk-taking and self-harming behaviors.

*L*ook for the loss.
Unresolved grief and
complicated bereavement are
too often overlooked by
doctors and therapists.

*O*ffer role playing in your therapy sessions. Take turns being the patient.

*A*sk your patients to supply factual evidence for what they think, feel and observe. This will allow them to identify cognitive distortions in stressful situations.

*I*f the patient tells a joke, laugh if it's funny and not self-depreciating. Then find the meaning.

The Process

Warn your patients well in advance of pending absence due to illness or pregnancy. Help them explore their anger, concern and anxiety about your health and your being away.

Zero in on specific interpersonal exchanges or "relationship episodes." These reveal much about your patient's wishes, anxieties and defenses.

Question. Confront. Clarify.

Interpret.

*T*he concept of "the inner child" has been overexposed and misused. Nonetheless, your patients may find compassion more readily for the children they were than for the adults they are.

❦

*U*sing the cognitive "downward arrow" technique, help your patient paint an absolute worst-case scenario for specific day-to- day anxieties. Repeatedly ask, "If that happened, what would result?" until you reach a central fear or core belief they have about themselves.

*T*he technique of prescribing the symptom is powerful but dangerous. Use paradox with great care.

*A*sk yourself after every session whether "work got done." Avoid becoming chatty, complacent or too comfortable. Did you listen carefully? Were you rigorous and systematic in your interventions? Ask yourself whether new insights emerged in the session. Use the word <u>work</u> with your patients and ask them regularly for perceptions of change and progress.

*W*arning: Have you and your patient formed a mutual admiration society?

*B*e suitably cautious about quick transformations and sudden cures, but don't dismiss rapid, healthy change as "a flight into health."

*H*ow would you and your patients know if they were getting better? What are specific signs and indicators along the way? Describe these together.

*C*ongratulate informed and thoughtful dissent.

*W*ould you describe your office as a safe place and a healing environment? Would your patient?

*W*hen assessing couples, look for the balance of power regarding education, money, childcare, chores, in-laws, sex and self-esteem.

*Y*our patient has four options in any situation: 1) leave; 2) change; 3) adapt; or 4) re-frame

*E*ncourage your patients to surround themselves with people who support their goals.

The Process

*D*on't let racist, sexist or homophobic remarks pass unchallenged. Find a way to interpret underlying fears or misconceptions without correcting or preaching.

*L*ook out for the "doorknob phenomenon." This is when charged details, "hot" topics are revealed by the patient in the last moments of the session. Gently interpret this pattern if the patient keeps introducing topics too late to deal with them.

"*I* know something I won't tell." Explore and interpret reasons that a patient introduces partial information but not the whole story. Often such coyness is about attempting to control or tantalize you or to test your real interest in caring and "discovering the truth."

*D*o not underestimate the role of money for either of you, in your work with a patient.

The Process

*F*our stages of "working through":
1) Gaining of a new insight
2) Application of the new insight
3) Conceiving oneself differently because of the insight
4) Mourning the loss of the old self, and severing
   relationships which reinforce old, maladaptive patterns.

*W*hen your patient visits his family of origin for holidays,
ask him to be a detective or observer, not a therapist.

*M*ake even your first assessment a therapeutic experience for the patient. One encounter may actually be enough or all the patient can afford right now.

The Process

*T*ermination takes at least four sessions. The pending goodbye in all forms of therapy produces intense feelings in most patients. Old losses and departures may be reawakened. Feelings of sadness, relief, anger, gratitude, disappointment may all emerge in the final phase of therapy. Make sure that you prepare for termination well in advance.

*T*wo key cognitive themes: help your patient explore doubts and struggles about competency and lovability.

*P*art of therapy is play. Leave

room for laughter.

The Process

*D*on't be afraid to use the words "love" and "hate" in your work.

*W*hen exploring the many hazards of the past, remind your patient of the here and now, and of choices they have at this moment.

*A*llow your patients to begin the session and set their own agendas and pace of discourse. This encourages autonomy right from the start.

*T*wo rules: 1) Do not chastise

2) Do not advise

The Process

$\mathcal{A}$ handshake, touch on a shoulder or hug may be powerful and therapeutic. They are nonetheless interventions and must be selected consciously by the therapist at the right moment.

$\mathcal{T}$hink of projection as a piece of clothing. If it doesn't fit, comment but don't wear it.

The Process

$\mathcal{A}$ good frame makes for good therapy. It is related to the articulated contract about personal boundaries, appointments, lateness, holidays, session length and other rules that govern the therapist-patient relationship and behavior. A well-defined frame helps to make each session a safe, reliable place for your patient and for you, especially when the emotional work gets stormy or chaotic.

$\mathcal{H}$elp your patient find the middle ground between all or nothing.

The Process

*A*ll therapies have these phases:
1) The Beginning—which is about building a working alliance and trust
2) The Middle—where the work gets done
3) The End—which is about negotiating the goodbye

A pause in therapy may be good for you, your patient, and the work. Do not leave things hanging, however. Describe how and when the next contact is to be made.

Seek out these three
key existential fears:
abandonment, engulfment,
annihilation.

The Process

*H*ave you discussed forgiving as a therapeutic option with your patient?

❧

*I*nquire about stillness. Invite your patients to be introspective and silent. Teach them how to sit with feeling and to do nothing.

❧

*R*egarding gifts: Be gracious when a patient offers you a present, but always gently explore what it means.

*T*he analysis of defense mechanisms is not obsolete. Provide your patients with a list and definitions of psychic defenses, and of cognitive errors or distortions. Invite them to be "on the lookout" in specific situations and to name the defense used.

❧

*W*elcome criticism and dissent. You may be the first person in this patient's life to allow it.

Replace the "shoulds" with
"coulds."

PRACTICAL TIPS

The Process

*I*f spoken words fail, try photographs, drawings, film, poetry or music to get your patient talking again.

*Y*our waiting room sends messages. Make it peaceful, beautiful, hospitable to all. Provide pamphlets and resource information so that learning takes place, even while the patient is waiting.

*B*uy yourself a very good chair. Your lower back will thank you ten years from now.

Practical Tips

When ending a contract prematurely, discharge your duty ethically and in a sound medicolegal fashion. Never drop a patient. Offer to transfer care to a colleague.

Try to offer your patients appointments for the same day and time each week. This ensures attendance and fosters a sense of safety and belonging.

*D*on't bother to tell your patients something they've heard a thousand times.

Practical Tips

*D*uring your assessment, ask your patients to describe both of their parents in three words. Much will be revealed.

*W*ith adolescents, never take the alliance for granted. Recreate it in every session.

*P*eople in a hurry cannot feel. Remind your patient to slow down. Remind yourself.

Self-help groups are a good source of support and can be a useful adjunct to therapy. Ask your patients about their experiences in the group to ensure that they are not receiving conflicting messages from you.

Do not fail to diagnose a learning disorder, hyperactivity or attention deficit. These continue to impair functioning throughout adulthood and are too often missed by therapists.

Practical Tips

When uncertain about cognitive functioning, diagnosis or personality structure, refer for neuropsychological testing.

Consider charging for missed sessions not due to emergencies. This may add concrete seriousness to your patient's view of the work.

When working with couples, frequently ask each member to paraphrase what the other is saying.

*D*esign specific homework tasks with your patients. Be
creative. Problem-solve and record outcomes around
these experiments. Changes in behavior may enable insight
to follow.

*D*o not eat or drink in a session, unless you plan to serve
your patients something. Then ask yourself why you're
both so hungry.

Practical Tips

*A*sk your patients to summarize key points at the end of a session and then to revisit them next time.

*I*f the therapy is stuck, revisit you patients' main goals and break them down into small, specific, workable pieces.

*H*elp your patient to see the difference between "sad" and "depressed." One is a feeling, the other an illness.

Practical Tips

*I*f medication is recommended for your patients while in therapy, explore the meaning of the drug for them. Does it represent failure, loss of control, dependence, denial, flight, or hope and enhancement with respect to therapy?

*I*f your patients' symptoms are complex compromises between two choices or two poles, describe the options.

Practical Tips

*F*ind out about the most traumatic event in your patients' lives. Were they trapped and terrified? Could they be suffering from bona fide post-traumatic stress disorder?

*A*s you contract together at the start of therapy, ask your patients to sign a "no-show" policy regarding cancellations and missed sessions. This emphasizes that both of you are protecting your hour together.

Practical Tips

*I*nquire about the well-being of your patients' children. Could your depressed or overwhelmed patients be neglecting or abusing them? Find out and intervene when necessary.

*P*revent rather than cure. Intervene early and quickly with acute trauma.

*D*on't assess the quality of a marriage or friendship by its duration. Find out how intimate it is.

*U*nless it's an emergency, do
not take telephone calls
during your patient's
session.

Practical Tips

*A*sk about safer sex. Many therapists take a sexual history during the intake session with the patient but do not ask subsequently about acting-out behaviors that might predispose the patient to contracting HIV or other STD's. Your role here is preventive, not authoritarian, and it may save your patient's life.

*T*hink twice before treating the friends, family members, spouses, or ex-partners of current patients. It's not impossible, only exponentially more difficult.

Practical Tips

*D*on't be late. If you are, ask yourself: Why now? Why with this client? Then apologize. Don't assume the person can make up the time. Avoid sending the message that your time is more valuable than your patients', that you get to be late and they don't, or that you both can be late.

*K*now your community resources—self-help groups, shelters, housing, job retraining programs. Your patients won't get better if they can't feed their families or find a job.

So much depends on two chairs. Pay attention to the furniture and decor in your office. Is your chair the same height as your client's? More comfortable? Do you sit away from your desk? Does the patient have a choice of where to sit? These cues send messages about comfort, authority and equality.

Remember to ask about the well siblings of sick children. They often suffer in silence.

*T*ake your time assessing the patient so that you know what it is you're offering and to whom.

*D*o not collude with a patient's request to cheat an insurance or drug plan. It will come back to haunt you and compromise the integrity of the work.

*M*ost people work best with deadlines. Introduce some element of goal-setting and time into the work, even if your approach is open-ended. This also promotes patients using time limits in life in a constructive manner.

Practical Tips

*T*owards the end of therapy, ask your patients how they plan to keep working on themselves and their lives. Be specific.

*F*our writing exercises: 1) Ask your patients to write a letter to the person they love most; 2) Ask your patients to write a letter to the person they love least; 3) Ask your patients to write their own obituary if they were to die tomorrow; and 4) Ask your patients what they would like to be able to write in their obituary if they died in five years.

Practical Tips

*I*f, on assessment, the patients' motivation to work is low, ask them to wait and come back when there is a sense of urgency or real commitment to make change.

❦

*T*ape record yourself, then listen. No matter how seasoned a therapist you are, get your patient's permission to tape record a session. You have already listened to what the patient said, this time listen to your own interventions. Are they useful, timely, precise? Could they be better delivered?

Practical Tips

*F*ind out what your secretary is doing. Patients form a relationship with the staff in your office as they wait for you. Make sure your receptionist is warm, discreet and patient, but not offering advice or attempting to do your job in between appointments!

*T*o preserve confidentiality, discuss with your patients how they can be reached between sessions and if, how and where messages can be left.

Practical Tips

*I*n brief therapy, keep the door open for re-consultation down the road, but don't mention this option until the very last session. Otherwise you may undermine the useful anxiety produced by pending termination.

❦

*I*f a former patient calls or writes, always respond promptly. This is basic to good manners and professionalism. It may also allow you to offer reinforcement, reassurance or a timely preventive intervention.

Practical Tips

*I*f you use an answering machine in your office, provide explicit instructions about confidentiality, when you will return calls, and what to do if the call is urgent and you're not available. Make sure your voice and message convey warmth, professionalism and respect.

*A*ssess the therapeutic contract on a regular basis, such as monthly. Revisit the presenting problem, the central focus, and goals and specify the gains made.

*M*ake use of simple rating scales from "one to ten" to help your patients to specify feelings, progress, convictions, and mood/anxiety states. They allow helpful comparisons over time.

Practical Tips

*I*f they look too thin, they are too thin. Ask about eating disorders.

*C*onsider offering a therapeutic "trial" of four sessions, rather than committing to a full contract. This allows assessment of "fit" between you and the patient, and of therapeutic alliance. It also allows you both to "bow out gracefully" if you can't help the patient.

When using DSM, don't forget Axis IV. It's the part about the real world.

Practical Tips

*H*elp your patients find a meaningful word, phrase, mantra or image that can be used in times of stress or isolation.

*I*f your patients are admitted to the hospital, call, visit or write to them on the ward. It will comfort them greatly.

*D*on't forget basic behaviorism. Reward and punishment actually work.

Practical Tips

*D*elineate the limits of confidentiality with each patient. Explain how you must proceed if there is evidence of potential harm to self or others in what the patient tells you.

*I*f you are late for a session, offer to make up the time during that session or at a later date. If the patient is late, you may choose to extend the hour but you are not obliged to do so.

*P*revent, where possible. Act, when necessary. A client's manic episode, impulsive or self-destructive gesture may destroy a career or family.

*T*hink twice before treating patients with no structure in their lives: no job, no studies, no volunteering, no routine, no outward pursuit. Therapy is not meant to be a full-time occupation or preoccupation.

Practical Tips

*Y*ou may choose to accept telephone calls or written communications from your patient's friends, family or work place. Specify beforehand to third parties that you will share the information with your patient. Never agree to keep secrets—they will paralyze the work.

*B*eware of splitting. Beware of triangles. You may not know that you've taken sides until it's too late!

Practical Tips

*D*on't neglect the body in the midst of all the words. Make certain that medical care is up-to-date. Teach your client proper breathing, relaxation, and self-soothing exercises. Refer for body work such as massage or yoga when appropriate.

*E*ncourage the reading of poetry, fiction and nonfiction during therapy. Prepare a list of books and articles that explore themes relevant to your patient's exploration.

Practical Tips

*T*he way you end a session may be as important as what happened during it. "We have to stop" or looking at your watch may be jarring to some patients. With each individual, find the language that reflects both the empathic and practical demands of ending the session. You don't have to be the master of the hour. Let your patients have visual access to a clock so they know when to stop themselves. Consider saying, "Let's continue next time," which sends a message of ongoing relationship rather than severance.

Practical Tips

*W*hen the patient asks you a question:
1) You may answer the question when you know what it really means
2) You may answer the question first providing you seek out what it means

*Y*ou will never regret taking a good developmental history.

*T*herapy 101: Start with open-ended questions.

Practical Tips

*U*nless it's an absolute emergency, never treat a friend, social acquaintance or family member. The therapeutic frame and boundaries are too shaky from the start.

*W*hen a patient misuses substances, tackle the drugs and alcohol first. Then offer therapy.

Practical Tips

*A*pply systems theory to the patients you care for. What roles are they fulfilling in their families, communities, corporations? Where are they in the pecking order? What would happen if they actually changed?

*A*sk about secrets, new and old, personal and familial, at home and at work. Now untie the knots of shame, one by one.

Practical Tips

*E*licit a central goal, theme, pattern or focus. Then revisit it in every session. Gently focus and re-focus.

*R*egarding taking notes in a session: Listen now, write later.

*P*rovide feedback on what you see as well as what you hear. You are a mirror for facial expressions, eye contact, body language, movement, and choice of dress.

*D*efine the number of minutes in the therapy hour, then don't waiver. The patient always knows when you're cheating.

Practical Tips

*B*e very sure that your patients' problem is not depression, mania, psychosis or a brain tumor. If in doubt, arrange a medical consultation at once.

*D*iscuss how you and your patient will behave should you meet socially. Always explore the event after it happens. Your own internal reactions to encountering a patient reveal much about your comfort with yourself.

*W*hen a person comes asking for therapy, ask "Why now?" Motivation and timing are everything.

Practical Tips

*T*ransference interpretations work wonders. They get to the heart of the matter, here and now.

❦

*T*hink twice before listing your home phone number in the telephone directory. Discuss your decision with your family or housemates.

❦

*B*arring emergencies, always get written permission before speaking to a third party or sending written records.

Practical Tips

$\mathcal{K}$eep pace with changes in mental health law in your area. Laws on commitment, reporting danger to a third party, and confidentiality are sometimes challenged and revised.

$\mathcal{K}$eep a small up-to-date confidential list of patient's names and phone numbers with you. You never know when you'll have to call a patient or re-book a session.

Practical Tips

*R*emind your patient to use simple techniques such as writing a "Pros and Cons" list when making important decisions.

*T*wo behavioral techniques to try with obsessional patients:
1) Thought stopping or shouting "stop" when intrusive thoughts emerge; 2) Have patients "snap" an elastic band with their wrist when obsessions start to preoccupy them.

Practical Tips

Send stoned or drunk patients home, but offer another appointment.

❧

Ask permission to record patients who talk too much. Then have them listen to the tape.

❧

Invite your patients to ask themselves this question: What would nine out of ten people feel in my situation?

Practical Tips

*R*emember to congratulate. Perseverance, gains, and realized goals should be duly noted with much encouragement.

THE ART

*D*iagnosis kills narrative. Don't slot people's stories into your DSM boxes. Listen respectfully.

*D*on't suppress your own personality when doing psychotherapy. Use it joyfully so that it doesn't get in the way.

*D*iscover where your patients find beauty in their lives.

Strive to be a healer, not a technician.

The Art

Always admit when you don't know something and when you're wrong. Doing so models openness, fallibility and vulnerability.

If a poet ignores grammar and structure intentionally, it's art. If it's ignored accidentally, it's an accident, even if successful. The same can be said of use or misuse of guidelines for therapy.

The Art

$\mathcal{P}$lay with reality. Look for multiple perspectives and the way you and your patient construct what is real.

❣

$\mathcal{T}$he best teacher of psychotherapy is a good personal therapy.

❣

$\mathcal{T}$here are many truths. Select those that are healing and constructive when choosing your formulations and interventions.

*H*elp patients experience gratitude as well as disappointment.

*T*here are, in essence, two emotional states: love and fear.

*B*efore giving an important interpretation that your patients may not want to hear, enlist their interest and ask their permission.

*J*ust because you've asked a
question once does not mean
that you have the answer.

The Art

When listening to the patient's story, don't mistake meaning for truth, or truth for meaning.

Love + Work = Happiness.

Part of what you do indirectly is to give permission for healthy strivings.

The Art

*I*t's never to late to change

*D*epending on timing and delivery, humor can hurt or heal.

*F*ind out who or what is your patient's God.

*P*eople in a hurry cannot feel. Remind your patients to slow down. Remind yourself.

The Art

You are like a modern priest, hearing confessions all day, but you may lack the power to absolve.

Use suspense as a way of sustaining your patient's interest and curiosity. Hint at key insights, allude to them in advance. A heightened arousal will foster learning and engagement in therapy.

*T*herapy is a lot like "dodge ball"—you dodge projections as you keep on playing.

❧

*E*licit the first, tiny step towards change. This is how the journey begins.

❧

*H*elp your patient rediscover a sense of proportion to tragedy and circumstance.

*P*reserve a healthy respect
for denial. It is there for a
good reason.

*I*n order to do psychotherapy, you'll need a basic theory of human development, defense mechanisms, the self, and psychopathology, which you're open to constantly revising. Otherwise you're merely stabbing in the dark.

*I*s there room for mystical experience in your theory? If not, what will you do when your patient has one?

*T*he patient needs to test you and to challenge limits in order to deepen trust. Remain patient and constant.

*I*magine the positive and negative ripple effects of your work with your patients, and the impact of changes they make in their lives.

*W*hen you're not sure what's going on, be kind rather than defensive.

The Art

*B*e constant in what you do, but don't become predictable in what you say. An element of surprise goes far in maximizing therapeutic impact.

*O*ne of your roles outside your office is to be an advocate for the mentally ill, to lessen their experience of social stigma and shame.

You are seldom helping only the patient in front of you. You are helping their partners, children, employees, and friends.

The Art

*L*ess is more. Even if your style is active or directive, keep your interventions brief, simple and unwordy. Monitor yourself. Are you talking too much? Interrupting? Asking too may questions? Are you dictating the agenda for each session? Let your patients bring what they want to explore that day and listen.

*M*any therapists feel that they haven't done their job if sadness and anger don't emerge in every session. Therapy is about all feelings, not just about suffering, so leave room for playfulness, joy and spontaneity!

The Art

*R*emember to ask about spirituality. Therapy is about "work, love and play," but add soul as a fourth dimension. This exploration need not involve traditional religion at all, but may cover existential concerns, the patients' search for greater meaning in their lives, and an untapped potential for joy.

*E*ncourage your patient and yourself to follow intuitions, to "Go with your gut." You may transcend technique and help your patient experience a breakthrough.

The Art

Words are drugs. Everything you say to a patient has the potential to help or harm. Your interventions need to be empathic, timely, and dispensed with care and the correct "dosing." An ill-timed, overly powerful interpretation or revelation could be as dangerous to the patient as a drug overdose.

Say "thank you" to your patients each time they teach you something, and when you say goodbye.

*D*on't forget to smile at your patients from time to time.

The Art

*I*f appropriate, encourage the use of ritual as part of healing: Writing a letter. Burning a letter. Keeping a journal. Saying a prayer. Constructing a small altar of symbols. Ritual may deepen meaning and promote understanding and change.

*R*emember, the Chinese figure for crisis is two symbols — danger and possibility.

*A*nswer this for yourself: Why do we suffer?

*T*herapy is like writing. Don't theorize. Show, don't tell.

The Art

What metaphor do you use to describe your work as a therapist: better a passenger than a driver, or better a midwife than a surgeon?

Don't fool yourself into thinking that you are neutral—you skillfully arrange inevitable conclusions.

Your job is to see the good in people.

*T*he drug you prescribe will
restore the imbalance in
the brain, not in the life.

The Art

*W*hen working with the chronically ill or dying patient, remember that change can happen quickly, and that hope and healing may not be the same thing as cure.

*T*hink of your most difficult patient as your teacher. In between curses and complaints, give thanks for what you've learned.

*R*emember: Resistance = fear.

The Art

*O*ne of your duties is to broker hope.

*L*earn to respect and follow your intuitions. You may transcend technique in that moment.

*A*fter you show your patients how to be assertive, remind them when to be silent.

The Art

You are not a witch-doctor or a wizard. If your client wants to know about the process of therapy—how it works, your techniques—provide explanation. What you do is at times mysterious, but it's not a secret.

Preoccupation with the past is regret. Preoccupation with the future is fantasy. What about now?

*K*eep the therapeutic space safe. All depends on trust.

*I*n and out of the session, let your patients sit with their feelings.

*L*earn from treatment failures, except don't call them that. You are not a failure, neither is your patient. Something, however small, likely happened in your work together.

The Art

*F*rom time to time read the artful language of your forebears. Even if you don't agree with the theories of Freud or Jung, you will see that they were not just technicians. They heard their patients' stories and found them beautiful.

*S*how the dependent person how to give, the independent person how to receive.

*Y*ou are mistaken if you think psychotherapy is not about morality, ethics, religion, politics, the law. Both you and your patient live in society.

*W*hat kind of friend are you to your patients? What kind of friend are your patients to themselves?

*R*espect silence. Learn to wait, not to fill in gaps. Take a deep breath. More often than not, important material emerges out of the reflective, frustrated, panicky or desolate feelings that accompany silence.

*H*ow reposed is your own countenance? How peaceful is the face that your patients see and sit before?

*T*he good therapist has slept well.

The Art

$\mathcal{Y}$ou are an alchemist. You turn dirt into gold.

$\mathcal{T}$here are always two people to take care of in any therapy session: the patient and the therapist.

$\mathcal{T}$he art of psychotherapy is ancient and honorable—don't let consumerism, research, technology or other agendas taint your exchange.

You are your patients'
advocate to themselves.
Resist being judge and jury.

The Art

*L*isten to your own voice: its tone, volume, quality, pitch. Your voice is your instrument. Tune it.

*C*reativity is not optional. Part of therapy is helping your patients find their passion, their bliss.

*W*hatever happens in or out of therapy, it's all grist for the mill.